BASIC NOTES IN PSYCHOPHARMACOLOGY

Previous books by the same author

Levi, M.I. (1987). MCQs for the MRCPsych Part I. (Lancaster: MTP Press)

Levi, M.I. (1988). MCQs for the MRCPsych Part II. (Lancaster: Kluwer Academic Publishers)

Levi, M.I. (1988). SAQs for the MRCPsych Part II. (Lancaster: Kluwer Academic Publishers)

Levi, M.I. (1989). Basic notes in psychiatry. (Lancaster: Kluwer Academic Publishers). Revised edition 1992

Levi, M.I. (1992). PMPs for the MRCPsych Part II. (Lancaster: Kluwer Academic Publishers)

Basic Notes in Psychopharmacology

by

Dr Michael I. Levi MB BS MRCPsych
Senior Registrar to the Professorial Unit of Psychiatry, Royal South Hants Hospital, Southampton, UK

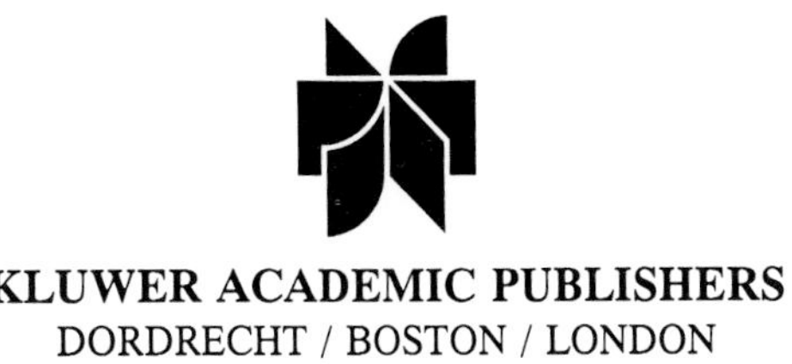

KLUWER ACADEMIC PUBLISHERS
DORDRECHT / BOSTON / LONDON

Distributors

for the United States and Canada: Kluwer Academic Publishers, PO Box 358, Accord Station, Hingham, MA 02018-0358, USA
for all other countries: Kluwer Academic Publishers Group, Distribution Center, PO Box 322, 3300 AH Dordrecht, The Netherlands

ISBN 0-7923-8806-2

A catalogue record for this book is available from the British Library.

Copyright

Published in the United Kingdom by Kluwer Academic Publishers, PO Box 55, Lancaster, UK.

Kluwer Academic Publishers BV incorporates the publishing programmes of D. Reidel, Martinus Nijhoff, Dr W. Junk and MTP Press.

Printed in Great Britain by Martins Ltd., Berwick on Tweed.

Contents

Foreword

Psychopharmacology is a rapidly developing subject, and an increasingly important one for the practising clinician. Powerful new approaches to the drug treatment of psychiatric disorders have evolved. With these new treatments come new side-effects and drug interactions, and it is ever more important that clinicians are aware of both the therapeutic opportunities and their associated hazards. The pace of change in this field makes it difficult for standard textbooks to keep up. Dr Levi is to be congratulated on producing a succinct guide to a complex and rapidly changing subject, which may guide supplemental further reading. This short text will act as both an excellent introduction to the subject, and a useful revision aid. Psychopharmacology is one aspect of psychiatry which lends itself particularly to examination by multiple choice questions, and this book is warmly recommended to trainee psychiatrists about to sit examinations. General practitioners, other physicians and surgeons, and other professionals allied to medicine will find the text broad in scope and up-to-date. Consultant psychiatrists (and examiners) may also discover new facts in these pages!

Robert Peveler, MA DPhil BM BCh MRCPsych
Senior Lecturer in Psychiatry
University of Southampton

October 1992

Introduction

The purpose of writing this book is to provide a concise summary of psychopharmacology in the form of notes. The drugs discussed in this book are those considered by the author to be the most important drugs that the practising physician needs to know about. The aim is to provide the principal mode of action, indications and adverse effects of the drugs covered. I have based these notes on what is generally regarded to be the most comprehensive textbook[1] for the MRCPsych examination. These notes represent my own view of current clinical practice.

The book is intended to have wide readership - particularly among junior hospital psychiatrists, general practitioners and medical students. In addition, the book will also be useful to psychiatric nurses, psychiatric social workers, psychiatric occupational therapists and clinical psychologists.

Reference

1. Kendell RE, Zealley AK, eds. Companion to psychiatric studies, fourth edition. 1988: Churchill Livingstone.

CHAPTER 1

Hypnotic and Anxiolytic Drugs

I. BENZODIAZEPINES

a) Mode of action

GABA (γ-aminobutyric acid) agonists; act at benzodiazepine receptors (BZ_1 and BZ_2) which are located postsynaptically throughout the brain at GABA-ergic synapses.

b) Indications

1. Transient insomnia in those who normally sleep well – if a benzodiazepine is indicated, use one that has a short half-life with little or no hangover effect and only prescribe one or two doses of the drug, e.g. lormetazepam; dose range 0.5 mg nocte to 1.5 mg nocte.

2. Anxiety neuroses – provide symptomatic relief of severe anxiety in the short term (should not be prescribed for more than 2–4 weeks), e.g. diazepam; dose range 2 mg t.d.s. increased if necessary to 15–30 mg daily in divided doses. The use of an antidepressant drug should also be considered in this situation (see later).

3. Phobic anxiety neuroses – provide some immediate relief of phobic symptoms in the short term.

4. Obsessive compulsive disorders – provide some short-term symptomatic relief (should not be prescribed for more than 2–4 weeks duration).

5. Acute organic disorder:

    i) May be used during the night-time to help the patient sleep.

    ii) In the special case of hepatic failure – may be used during the daytime to calm the patient despite their sedative effects, since they are less likely to precipitate coma – cf. haloperidol (which is the usual drug of choice to calm such patients).

    iii) In the special case of alcohol withdrawal – chlordiazepoxide is the most suitable drug.

6. Chronic organic disorder – may be used to alleviate anxiety.

7. Barbiturate dependence – used to cover the withdrawal symptoms from barbiturates.

8. Acutely disturbed behaviour – if an antipsychotic drug alone fails to bring the situation under control, they may be given in addition to this, e.g. a slow intravenous injection of 4 mg of lorazepam, if necessary repeated every 2 hours until the patient settles.

c) Adverse effects

1. Both psychic and physical dependence occur.

2. Chronic benzodiazepine dependence – often manifests features of benzodiazepine intoxication which are:

    i) Unsteadiness of gait.
    ii) Dysarthria.

iii) Drowsiness.
iv) Nystagmus.

3. Withdrawal effects from benzodiazepines:

   i) Rebound insomnia.
   ii) Tremor.
   iii) Anxiety.
   iv) Restlessness.
   v) Appetite disturbance.
   vi) Weight loss.
   vii) Sweating.
   viii) Convulsions.
   ix) Confusion.
   x) Toxic psychosis.
   xi) A condition resembling delirium tremens.

4. Benzodiazepines – cf. barbiturates. Features of benzodiazepines:

   i) Less side-effects – including less risk of respiratory depression.
   ii) Less severe physical dependence.
   iii) Less dangerous in overdosage.
   iv) Less likely to interact with other drugs – as induction of hepatic microsomal enzymes does not occur.

II. BARBITURATES

a) Mode of action

GABA agonists; do not act at benzodiazepine receptors; may have specific binding sites elsewhere on the neuronal membrane.

b) Indications

1. Severe intractable insomnia in patients already taking barbiturates – even in such patients, an attempt to withdraw the barbiturate should be considered, covering the withdrawal syndrome with a benzodiazepine.

2. Hysteria – classically, abreaction was brought about by an intravenous injection of small amounts of amylobarbitone sodium. In the resulting state, the patient is encouraged to relive the stressful events that provoked the hysteria, and to express the accompanying emotions. Now, such abreaction can be initiated more safely by a slow intravenous injection of 10 mg of diazepam.

c) Adverse effects

1. Both psychic and physical dependence occur.

2. Chronic barbiturate dependence – often manifests features of barbiturate intoxication which are:

   i) Slurred speech.
   ii) Incoherence.
   iii) Dullness.
   iv) Drowsiness.
   v) Nystagmus.
   vi) Depression.

3. Withdrawal effects from barbiturates:

   i) Clouding of consciousness.
   ii) Disorientation.
   iii) Hallucinations.

iv) Major seizures.
v) Anxiety.
vi) Restlessness.
vii) Pyrexia.
viii) Tremulousness.
ix) Insomnia.
x) Hypotension.
xi) Nausea.
xii) Vomiting.
xiii) Anorexia.
xiv) Twitching.
xv) A condition resembling delirium tremens.

4. Drug interactions – induction of hepatic microsomal enzymes leads to increased metabolism of:

i) The oral contraceptive pill.
ii) Corticosteroids.
iii) Warfarin.
iv) Tricyclic antidepressants.

III. CHLORAL DERIVATIVES

a) Mode of action

GABA agonists.

b) Indications

Short-term treatment of insomnia, particularly in the elderly, e.g. chloral hydrate; usual dose range 0.5 g nocte to 1 g nocte taken with plenty of water (should not be prescribed for more than 1–2 weeks duration).

c) Adverse effects

Triclofos sodium causes fewer gastrointestinal disturbances cf. chloral hydrate.

IV. OTHERS

1. CHLORMETHIAZOLE

a) Mode of action

GABA agonist.

b) Indications

In the management of alcohol withdrawal for inpatients only, chlormethiazole may be prescribed in either of two ways:

1. On an as-required basis, i.e. flexibly according to the patient's symptoms.

2. On a reducing regime basis, i.e. on a fixed 6-hourly regime of gradually decreasing dosage over 6–9 days. *N.B. Alternatively, chlordiazepoxide may be used in the management of alcohol withdrawal – this has the advantage over chlormethiazole of being less addictive and being less dangerous if taken in combination with alcohol.*

c) Adverse effects

May cause acute cardiac arrest or acute respiratory arrest if taken in combination with alcohol.

2. β-BLOCKERS

a) Mode of action

Block β-adrenoreceptors in the heart, peripheral vasculature, bronchi, liver and pancreas.

b) Indications

Limited use in treating anxiety neuroses in which palpitations, sweating or tremor are the most troublesome symptoms, i.e. those anxiety neuroses with predominantly somatic symptoms, e.g. propanolol; dose range 40 mg b.d. to 40 mg t.d.s.
N.B. β-Blockers have little effect on subjective feelings of anxiety.

c) Adverse effects

Contraindicated in patients with:

1. Asthma.
2. A history of obstructive airways disease.
3. Uncontrolled heart failure.
4. Second- or third-degree heart block.

3. BUSPIRONE

a) Mode of action

1. Thought to act at specific serotonin ($5HT_{1A}$) receptors.
2. Response to treatment may take up to 2 weeks – similar to antidepressant drugs.

b) Indications

1. Limited use in short-term treatment of chronic anxiety neuroses; usual dose range 5 mg t.d.s. to 10 mg t.d.s.

2. May yet turn out to be an effective antidepressant.

c) Adverse effects

1. Physical dependence and abuse liability not yet established.

2. Since this is a newly introduced drug for the treatment of anxiety, caution should be adopted and the drug should only be prescribed in the short-term.

4. ZOPICLONE

a) Mode of action

1. The first cyclopyrrolone.

2. GABA agonist – although not a benzodiazepine, it acts at benzodiazepine receptors (BZ_1 and BZ_2) which are located postsynaptically throughout the brain at GABA-ergic synapses.

b) Indications

1. Transient insomnia in those who normally sleep well – as an alternative to a benzodiazepine; dose range 7.5 mg nocte to 15 mg nocte.

2. For short-term use only (preferably only 1 or 2 doses).

c) Adverse effects

Since it acts at benzodiazepine receptors, it may give rise to the problems of physical dependence as observed in benzodiazepines if used for long-term treatment.

CHAPTER 2

Antipsychotic Drugs

CLASSIFICATION

1. Phenothiazines:

    i) Aliphatic (chlorpromazine).
    ii) Piperidine (thioridazine).
    iii) Piperazine (trifluoperazine/fluphenazine).

2. Butyrophenones (haloperidol/droperidol).

3. Thioxanthenes (flupenthixol/zuclopenthixol).

4. Diphenylbutylpiperidines (pimozide/fluspirilene).

5. Substituted benzamides (sulpiride/remoxipride).

6. Dibenzoxazepines (clozapine).

I. CHLORPROMAZINE

a) Mode of action

1. Dopamine antagonist; blocks D_2 receptors in the mesolimbic cortical bundle – which mediates the antipsychotic action of chlorpromazine.

2. It also has several other biochemical actions which mediate the side-effects of chlorpromazine:

    i) Dopamine blocking activity at other sites (see later).

- ii) Anti-adrenergic activity (i.e. α-adrenoreceptor blocking activity).
- iii) Anticholinergic activity.
- iv) Antiserotonergic activity.
- v) Antihistaminergic activity.

b) Indications

1. Personality disorders – may be given for short periods at times of unusual stress.

2. Obsessive compulsive disorders – small doses of value when anxiolytic treatment is needed for more than the 2–4 weeks duration that benzodiazepines are prescribed for.

3. Simple paranoid state – symptoms are sometimes relieved.

4. Affective disorders:

   - i) Control of the psychotic components of psychotic depression.
   - ii) Usually brings the symptoms of acute mania under rapid control.

5. Schizophrenia:

   - i) Control and maintenance therapy in schizophrenia.
   - ii) Chlorpromazine is more sedative and causes less extrapyramidal side-effects of haloperidol – thus, chlorpromazine is the drug of choice for schizophrenia.

6. Chronic organic disorder – alleviation of certain symptoms of dementia:

   i) Anxiety.
   ii) Overactivity.
   iii) Delusions.
   iv) Hallucinations.

   N.B. Care is needed to find the optimal dose.

7. Behavioural disturbances – tranquillization and emergency control.

8. Severe anxiety – short-term adjunctive treatment.

9. Terminal disease.

10. Anti-emetic.

11. Intractable hiccup.

c) Side-effects

1. Extrapyramidal side-effects (EPSE) – mediated by dopamine blocking activity at D_2 receptors in the nigrostriatal pathway:

   i) Acute dystonic reactions.
   ii) Akathisia.
   iii) Pseudoparkinsonism.
   iv) Tardive dyskinesia.

2. Anti-adrenergic side-effects:

   i) Postural hypotension.
   ii) Failure of ejaculation.
   iii) Sedation.

3. Anticholinergic side-effects:

    i) Dry mouth.
    ii) Blurred vision.
    iii) Constipation.
    iv) Urinary retention.
    v) Tachycardia.
    vi) Impotence.

4. Antiserotonergic side-effect – depression.

5. Antihistaminergic side-effect: sedation.
   N.B. Sedation is mainly mediated through anti-adrenergic activity.

6. Hyperprolactinaemia – mediated by dopamine blocking activity at D_2 receptors in the tubero-infundibular system – galactorrhoea in both women and men.

7. Impaired temperature regulation:

    i) Hypothermia.
    ii) Hyperpyrexia.

8. Neuroleptic malignant syndrome (NMS).

9. Bone marrow suppression – leucopenia.

10. Skin photosensitivity and pigmentation.

11. Cardiac arrhythmias.

12. Cholestatic jaundice.

13. Seizures (due to lowering of the convulsive threshold).

14. Weight gain.

II. HALOPERIDOL

a) Mode of action

1. Greater dopamine blocking activity
2. Less anti-adrenergic activity
3. Less anti-cholinergic activity

} cf. chlorpromazine.

b) Indications

Drug of choice for:

1. Mania.
2. Treatment of acute organic disorder during the daytime.
3. Bringing acutely disturbed behaviour under immediate control – since it is less sedative and causes less postural hypotension than chlorpromazine.

c) Side-effects

1. More EPSE
2. Less sedation
3. Less postural hypotension
4. Less anticholinergic side-effects

} cf. chlorpromazine.

5. NMS – a particular problem with haloperidol if a daily dosage in excess of 20 mg q.d.s. is combined with lithium carbonate at a serum level of greater than 1.0 mmol/L.

III. DROPERIDOL

a) Mode of action

Similar to haloperidol.

b) Indications

1. Useful in manic patients who fail to respond to haloperidol.

2. Useful in agitated manic patients who require rapid calming.

c) Side-effects

Similar to haloperidol.

IV. TRIFLUOPERAZINE

a) Mode of action

1. Greater dopamine blocking activity
2. Less anti-adrenergic activity
3. Less anticholinergic activity

} cf. chlorpromazine.

b) Indications

1. Useful in psychotic patients where sedation is undesirable (i.e. retarded psychotic patients) – since it is less sedative – cf. chlorpromazine.

2. Useful in psychotic patients with intractable auditory hallucinations; usual dose range 5 mg b.d. to 5 mg t.d.s.

c) Side-effects

1. More EPSE
2. Less sedation
3. Less postural hypotension
4. Less anticholinergic side-effects

} cf. chlorpromazine.

V. THIORIDAZINE

a) Mode of action

1. Less dopamine blocking activity
2. Greater anti-adrenergic activity
3. Greater anticholinergic activity

} cf. chlorpromazine.

b) Indications

Particularly useful in elderly patients for psychotic symptoms and agitation (since less EPSE – cf. chlorpromazine).

c) Side-effects

1. Less EPSE
2. More sedation
3. More postural hypotension
4. More anticholinergic side-effects

} cf. chlorpromazine.

5. Retinitis pigmentosa – particularly induced by thioridazine.

VI. SULPIRIDE

a) Mode of action

1. Low doses – thought to block pre-synaptic dopamine autoreceptors (D_3 and D_4 receptors).

2. High doses – blocks post-synaptic dopamine receptors; more specific blocker of D_2 receptors – cf. D_1 receptors.

b) Indications

1. Low doses – alerting effect on schizophrenic patients with negative symptoms such as apathy and social withdrawal (optimum dosage 400 mg b.d.).

2. High doses – useful in schizophrenic patients with florid positive symptoms such as delusions and hallucinations (optimum dosage 800 mg b.d.).

c) Side-effects

1. Less EPSE – cf. chlorpromazine.

2. Less sedation – cf. chlorpromazine.

3. Tendency to cause galactorrhoea.

VII. PIMOZIDE

a) Mode of action

More specific blocker of D_1 and D_2 receptors – cf. chlorpromazine.

b) Indications

1. Useful in maintenance treatment of schizophrenic patients who will not comply with antipsychotic depot injections – because of its long half-life, it need only be taken once a day to prevent relapse of schizophrenia (dose range 2–20 mg daily).

2. Useful in monosymptomatic delusional psychosis – it is claimed that pimozide has success in specifically targeting monosymptomatic hypochondriacal delusions (dose range 4–16 mg daily).

c) Side-effects

1. Less EPSE
2. Less sedation

} cf. chlorpromazine.

3. Following reports of sudden unexplained death, CSM recommends:

   i) An ECG prior to commencing treatment in all patients.
   ii) ECGs at regular intervals in patients taking over 16 mg daily.
   iii) A review of the need for pimozide if arrhythmias develop.

VIII. CLOZAPINE

a) Mode of action

1. Less dopamine blocking activity
2. Greater anti-adrenergic activity
3. Greater anticholinergic activity

} cf. chlorpromazine.

b) Indications

The treatment of schizophrenia in patients unresponsive to, or intolerant of, conventional antipsychotic drugs; at least one drug from three chemically distinct classes should be given a full therapeutic trial before considering clozapine (see earlier classification of antipsychotic drugs); in addition, it may be worth considering a course of electroconvulsive therapy (ECT) before starting clozapine therapy, since this can be an effective treatment in resistant schizophrenia (particularly when a significant affective component is present).
N.B. Clozapine should only be used by psychiatrists.

c) Side-effects

1. Less EPSE
2. More sedation
3. More postural hypotension
4. More anticholinergic side-effects

} cf. chlorpromazine.

5. It causes agranulocytosis (life-threatening) in 2–3% of patients taking the drug – its use is therefore restricted to patients registered with the clozaril patient monitoring service (CPMS) whereby the patient has regular full blood counts to detect any possible agranulocytosis; should this occur, the clozapine must be stopped.

IX. REMOXIPRIDE

a) Mode of action

1. Highly selective blocker of D_2 receptors; in addition it has a regional preference for blocking D_2 receptors in the mesolimbic cortical bundle cf. the nigrostriatal pathway and the tubero-infundibular system.

2. Little or no affinity for D_1 receptors and other central neurotransmitter receptors.

b) Indications

1. Treatment of both the positive and negative symptoms of schizophrenia; it appears efficacious in treating both sets of symptoms equally well (dose range 300 mg – 600 mg daily).

2. Useful in maintenance treatment of schizophrenic patients who will not comply with antipsychotic depot injections – because of its sustained release nature, it need only be taken once a day to prevent relapse of schizophrenia.

3. Treatment of acutely disturbed behaviour; most usefully in conjunction with zuclopenthixol acetate.
   N.B. Remoxipride is only available as an oral preparation in the UK.

c) Adverse effects

1. Less EPSE cf. other antipsychotic drugs.

2. Few clinically relevant anti-adrenergic side-effects.

3. Few clinically relevant anticholinergic side-effects.

4. Little tendency to cause galactorrhoea (cf. sulpiride).

5. Does not appear to cause arrhythmias (cf. pimozide).

6. Appears to have a neutral psychomotor profile, being non-sedating and non-alerting in nature.

7. May impair liver function – therefore caution is advised in severe hepatic impairment, i.e. the starting dose should be 150 mg daily (this starting dose should also be used for patients with severe renal impairment and elderly patients).

IX. ANTIPSYCHOTIC DEPOT INJECTIONS

A. IN GENERAL

a) Mode of action

Long-acting depot injections administered intramuscularly as an oily injection and slowly released into the bloodstream.

b) Indications

1. For maintenance therapy of schizophrenia – more conveniently given than oral antipsychotic preparations ensuring better patient compliance.

2. For prophylaxis of bipolar affective disorder in patients who have poor compliance with oral prophylactic medication – depot medication certainly protects against hypomanic relapse and some clinicians believe it also protects against a subsequent depressive relapse.

c) Side-effects

1. They should always initially be given as a test dose injection to ensure that the patient does not experience undue side-effects or any idiosyncratic reactions to the medication.

2. They may give rise to a higher incidence of EPSE – cf. oral antipsychotic preparations.

B. MORE SPECIFICALLY

1. FLUPHENAZINE DECANOATE

a) Indications

1. Useful in treating agitated or aggressive schizophrenic patients.

2. May be useful for the control of aggressive patients (in view of its sedative nature).

b) Adverse effects

Contraindicated in severely depressed states – in view of its tendency to cause depression.

2. FLUPENTHIXOL DECANOATE

a) Indications

1. Useful in treating retarded or withdrawn schizophrenic patients – in view of its alerting nature.

2. May be the antipsychotic depot injection of choice in patients with bipolar affective disorder – since its mood elevating effect would certainly protect against depressive relapse.

b) Adverse effects

Not suitable for the treatment of agitated or aggressive schizophrenic patients – since it can cause over-excitement in such patients in view of its alerting nature.

3. ZUCLOPENTHIXOL DECANOATE

a) Indications

1. Useful in treating agitated or aggressive schizophrenic patients.

2. May be useful for the control of aggressive patients (this specific indication is more clearly established for zuclopenthixol decanoate – cf. fluphenazine decanoate) – in view of its sedative nature (zuclopenthixol decanoate is more sedative than fluphenazine decanoate).

b) Adverse effects

Not suitable for the treatment of retarded or withdrawn schizophrenic patients – since it may exacerbate psychomotor retardation in such patients in view of its sedative nature.

4. ZUCLOPENTHIXOL ACETATE

a) Mode of action

Short-acting injection administered intramuscularly as an oily injection and rapidly released into the bloodstream.

b) Indications

Useful for immediate management of acutely disturbed behaviour as an alternative to haloperidol since:

1. Zuclopenthixol acetate is more sedative than haloperidol.

2. A short course of these injections (maximum of four) is more easily administered to the patient – cf. trying to persuade such a patient to comply with regular oral or intramuscular haloperidol.

c) Caution

Treatment duration should not exceed 2 weeks with a maximum dosage of 150 mg for each injection and a maximum dosage of 400 mg for each course of injections.

5. FLUSPIRILENE

a) Mode of action

Long-acting depot injection administered intramuscularly as an aqueous suspension and slowly released into the bloodstream – but with a shorter duration of action – cf. other antipsychotic depot injections.

b) Advantages

1. Probably decreased incidence of EPSE cf. other antipsychotic depot injections.

2. Administered to patient more easily (i.e. with less physical resistance at the site of injection) as it is given as an aqueous suspension – cf. other antipsychotic depot injections which are given as an oily injection.

c) Disadvantages

1. Needs to be administered once every week – cf. other antipsychotic depot injections which need to be administered generally less frequently (once every 2 weeks to once every 4 weeks).

2. May crystallize at the site of injection with prolonged use leading to tissue damage in the form of subcutaneous nodules (this may be offset somewhat by rotating the site of injection as often as possible).

CHAPTER 3

Antidepressant drugs

I. TRICYCLIC ANTIDEPRESSANTS (TCAs)

A. IN GENERAL

a) Mode of action

Monoamine re-uptake inhibitors (MARIs) – inhibit the re-uptake of both serotonin and noradrenaline into the pre-synaptic neurone, with the result that both neurotransmitters accumulate within the synapse. Such biochemical changes occur within several hours following administration of the drug, while the antidepressant action of the drug is delayed for about two weeks, indicating that some secondary process must be taking place.

b) Indications

1. Anxiety neuroses – when medication has to be prolonged beyond the few (2–4) weeks for which benzodiazepines are prescribed; effective due to their anxiolytic properties.

2. Phobic anxiety neuroses – again effective due to their anxiolytic properties.

3. Obsessive compulsive disorders – when anxiolytic treatment has to be prolonged beyond the few (2–4) weeks for which benzodiazepines are prescribed.

N.B. Clomipramine is claimed to have a specific anti-obsessional effect in addition to its anxiolytic effect (see later).

4. Hypochondriasis – some clinicians advocate a trial of TCAs in all patients (especially if the patient is depressed).

5. Affective disorders:

   i) Treatment of depressive disorders in the acute stage.
   ii) Preventing relapse of depressive disorders – need to continue medication for 6 months post-clinical recovery after the first episode of a unipolar affective disorder and for several (1–3) years post-clinical recovery after 2 or more episodes of a unipolar affective disorder.

6. Chronic organic disorder with depressive symptoms – a trial of antidepressant medication is worthwhile even in the presence of dementia.

7. Bulimia nervosa – TCAs produce an immediate reduction in binging and vomiting. However, their long-term effects are less pronounced.

c) Side-effects

1. Anticholinergic side-effects:

   i) Dry mouth.
   ii) Blurred vision.
   iii) Constipation.
   iv) Urinary retention.

v) Tachycardia.
vi) Impotence.
vii) Sweating.
viii) Confusion.
ix) Exacerbation of narrow angle glaucoma.

2. Cardiovascular side-effects (due to quinidine-like actions):

   i) Tachycardia.
   ii) Arrhythmias.
   iii) Postural hypotension.
   iv) Syncope.
   v) Cardiomyopathy.
   vi) Cardiac failure.
   vii) ECG changes (e.g. inversion and flattening of T waves).

3. Other side-effects:

   i) Seizures (due to lowering of the convulsive threshold).
   ii) Hypomania (in patients with bipolar affective disorder).
   iii) Tremor.
   iv) Weight gain.
   v) Agranulocytosis (uncommon).
   vi) NMS (rare).
   vii) Tardive dyskinesia (rare).

d) Toxic effects (i.e. effects of overdosage)

1. Cardiac arrhythmias/arrest.
2. Prolongation of the QRS complex.
3. Postural hypotension.

4. Epileptic seizures.
5. Hyperreflexia.
6. Mydriasis.
7. Coma.
8. Death.

B. MORE SPECIFICALLY

1. AMITRIPTYLINE

a) Indications

Treatment of agitated depression – in view of its sedative nature:

1. Starting dose – 75 mg nocte; build up gradually over 1–2 weeks to 150 mg nocte (usual dose required for efficacy in treating both the acute stage and for prophylaxis).

2. In patients unresponsive to 150 mg nocte – pushing the dose up to 225 mg nocte or even 300 mg nocte (maximum) may be clinically effective.

b) Adverse effects

Not suitable for the treatment of retarded depression – since it may exacerbate psychomotor retardation in such patients in view of its sedative nature.

2. IMIPRAMINE

a) Indications

1. Treatment of anxiety neuroses – imipramine may have a specific effect on autonomic reactivity in panic disorder (where the starting dose is 25 mg).

2. Treatment of phobic anxiety neuroses – some clinicians consider imipramine to be the treatment of choice in agoraphobia.

3. Treatment of retarded depression – in view of its alerting nature (similar dosage requirements as for amitriptyline – see earlier).

b) Adverse effects

Not suitable for the treatment of agitated depression – since it may cause over-excitement in such patients in view of its alerting nature.

3. DOTHIEPIN

a) Indications

Treatment of agitated depression – in view of its sedative nature:

1. Starting dose – 75 mg nocte, increased after 4 days to 150 mg nocte (similar dosage requirements as for amitriptyline – see earlier).

2. Particularly useful in treating elderly patients – since it has less anticholinergic side-effects and less cardiovascular side-effects – cf. amitriptyline (this also explains why the starting dose of dothiepin can be stepped up more quickly to the therapeutic dose – cf. amitriptyline).

b) Adverse effects

If taken in overdosage, dothiepin is the TCA most commonly responsible for deaths in the UK at present.

4. CLOMIPRAMINE

a) Mode of action

Inhibits the re-uptake of both serotonin and noradrenaline. However, it is a more selective inhibitor of the re-uptake of serotonin cf. the other TCAs.

b) Indications

1. Treatment of obsessive compulsive disorders – it has been reported that clomipramine has a specific action against obsessional symptoms (due to it being a more selective re-uptake inhibitor of serotonin cf. the other TCAs).

2. Treatment of agitated depression – in view of its sedative nature.

c) Side-effects

It has more anticholinergic side-effects and more cardiovascular side-effects – cf. amitriptyline – which may prevent some patients from tolerating it.

II. SECOND-GENERATION ANTIDEPRESSANTS

A. IN GENERAL

a) Definition

The next class of antidepressant drugs to be developed after TCAs.

b) Indications

Particularly useful in the following groups of depressed patients:

1. Patients intolerant of the side-effects of TCAs.
2. Elderly patients.
3. Patients at high risk of suicide.
4. Patients treated in the general practice setting.

c) Adverse effects

1. Less anticholinergic side-effects and less cardiovascular side-effects – cf. TCAs.

2. Safer in overdosage – cf. TCAs.

B. MORE SPECIFICALLY

1. LOFEPRAMINE

a) Mode of action

1. Mainly a noradrenergic re-uptake inhibitor, i.e. it is a relatively selective re-uptake inhibitor of noradrenaline.

2. Structurally a tricyclic antidepressant – however, its adverse effects profile is considerably different from the older 'parent' TCAs (see below).

b) Indications

Treatment and prophylaxis of retarded depression – in view of its alerting nature.

c) Adverse effects

1. Not suitable for the treatment of agitated depression – since it may cause over-excitement (e.g. sweating, palpitations) in such patients in view of its alerting nature.

2. Much improved side-effects profile – cf. older 'parent'

TCAs – i.e. lofepramine has fewer anticholinergic side-effects and less cardiotoxicity. Hence, more suitable for use in physically ill patients cf. older 'parent' TCAs.

3. Remarkable record of safety in overdosage – only three deaths recorded to date.

2. MIANSERIN

a) Mode of action

1. An α_2 pre-synaptic autoreceptor antagonist – a novel mode of action for an antidepressant drug with no significant effect on the re-uptake of monoamines (i.e. it is only a weak inhibitor of serotonin and noradrenaline re-uptake); despite this, it still appears to be an effective antidepressant.

2. Structurally a tetracyclic antidepressant.

b) Adverse effects

1. No anticholinergic side-effects
2. Minimal cardiotoxicity – safer in overdosage
3. Rarely causes convulsions – i.e. less proconvulsive

} cf. TCAs.

4. May cause agranulocytosis:

   i) A full blood count is recommended every 4 weeks during the first 3 months of treatment.

ii) If signs of infection develop (e.g. sore throat, fever, stomatitis), treatment should be stopped, a full blood count obtained and subsequent clinical monitoring should continue.

iii) This unfortunate side-effect of mianserin together with its questionable efficacy (see mode of action earlier) has limited the prescription of the drug in the hospital setting.

III. SELECTIVE SEROTONIN RE-UPTAKE INHIBITORS (SSRIs) (ALSO KNOWN AS 5-HT RE-UPTAKE INHIBITORS)

A. IN GENERAL

a) Definition

The next class of antidepressant drugs to follow the second-generation antidepressants in time, i.e. SSRIs are effectively ‘third-generation antidepressants’.

b) Mode of action

SSRIs are highly selective serotonin re-uptake inhibitors with little or no effect on noradrenergic processes.

c) Indications

1. Treatment of depressive disorders, particularly in:

   i) Patients intolerant of the side-effects of TCAs.

ii) Elderly patients.
iii) Patients with a high risk of suicide.
iv) Patients treated in the general practice setting.
v) Patients with cardiovascular disease.
vi) Patients with epilepsy – SSRIs are the least proconvulsive of all antidepressants, i.e. they are the least likely to lower the convulsive threshold.

2. Preventing relapse of depressive disorders – need to continue medication for 6 months post-clinical recovery after the first episode of a unipolar affective disorder and for several (1–3) years post-clinical recovery after 2 or more episodes of a unipolar affective disorder.

3. Treatment of panic disorder.

4. Treatment of obsessive compulsive disorder.

5. Treatment of aggressive behaviour.

6. Treatment of premenstrual syndrome (PMS).

7. Treatment of bulimia nervosa (fluoxetine – see later).

d) Adverse effects

1. No anticholinergic side-effects
2. No clinically significant cardiovascular side-effects
3. Safer in overdosage

} cf. TCAs.

4. Although SSRIs are thought to reduce both suicidal ideation and aggressive behaviour, some patients may have paradoxically increased suicidal ideation and increased aggressive behaviour.

B. MORE SPECIFICALLY

1. FLUVOXAMINE

The first SSRI introduced into the UK in 1987.

a) Mode of action

1. Structurally a monocyclic antidepressant.
2. No active metabolite.
3. 17–22 hour half-life.

b) Indications

Treatment of agitated depression – in view of its neutral psychomotor profile, i.e. it does not alert or sedate.

c) Adverse effects

1. High incidence of nausea and vomiting particularly during the first few days of treatment – this may prevent some patients from tolerating it; such gastrointestinal side-effects may be offset somewhat by taking tablets immediately after food and by initiating treatment at a dosage of 50 mg nocte for one week and then stepping it up to the usual therapeutic dosage of 50 mg b.d. (some patients may only respond to the higher therapeutic dosage of 100 mg b.d.).

2. Less suitable for the treatment of retarded depression – in view of its non-alerting nature.

3. Not suitable for patients with hepatic impairment – since it may elevate hepatic enzymes with symptoms.

2. FLUOXETINE

Introduced into the UK in 1989.

a) Mode of action

1. Structurally a bicyclic antidepressant.

2. Long half-life with an active metabolite (norfluoxetine) which itself has a long half-life with similar activity to the parent compound.

b) Indications

1. Treatment of retarded depression – in view of its alerting nature (dosage: 20 mg mane).

2. Treatment of bulimia nervosa (dosage: 60 mg mane).

3. Treatment of obsessive compulsive disorders – dose range: 20–80 mg mane; increasing the dosage within this range increasingly targets obsessional symptoms.

c) Adverse effects

1. Not suitable for the treatment of agitated depression – since it may cause over-excitement (e.g. sweating, palpitations) in such patients in view of its alerting nature.

2. Not suitable for patients with severe renal impairment – in view of its long half-life and active metabolite.

3. Not suitable for patients with severe weight loss – in view of its catabolic/anorectic nature.

4. Nausea and vomiting appear to be less of a problem with fluoxetine cf. fluvoxamine.

3. SERTRALINE

Introduced into the UK in 1990.

a) Mode of action

1. Structurally different from fluvoxamine, fluoxetine and paroxetine.

2. Has an active metabolite (desmethylsertraline) which has a long half-life with about one eighth of the activity of the parent compound.

b) Indications

1. Treatment of retarded depression – in view of its slightly alerting nature (dose range: 50 mg mane to 200 mg mane).

2. The only current SSRI to have a licence for the long-term maintenance treatment of depression.

c) Adverse effects

1. Not suitable for the treatment of agitated depression – since it may cause over-excitement (e.g. sweating, palpitations) in such patients in view of its slightly alerting nature.

2. Not suitable for patients with hepatic impairment – since it may elevate hepatic enzymes with symptoms.

3. Not suitable for patients with renal impairment – in view of its active metabolite.

4. Doses of more than 100 mg mane should not be used for more than eight weeks, which limits the usefulness of the drug in those patients requiring the higher dosing to break into their clinical depression.

4. PAROXETINE

Introduced into the UK in 1991.

a) Mode of action

1. Structurally different from fluvoxamine, fluoxetine and sertraline.

2. The most selective and most potent of all currently available SSRIs.

3. No active metabolite.

4. 24 hour half-life.

b) Indications

1. Treatment of agitated depression – in view of its neutral psychomotor profile, i.e. it does not alert or sedate (dosage: 20 mg mane; this may be increased up to 50 mg mane in adults by 10 mg increments if necessary).

2. Treatment of depression with associated anxiety – it is the only current SSRI to have a licence for this.

c) Adverse effects

1. Less suitable for the treatment of retarded depression – in view of its non-alerting nature.

2. Nausea and vomiting appear to be less of a problem with paroxetine cf. fluvoxamine.

3. The most suitable SSRI for patients with hepatic or renal impairment – although caution is still advised.

IV. MONOAMINE OXIDASE INHIBITORS (MAOIs)

a) Mode of action

Inhibit the enzyme monoamine oxidase which is present in the pre-synaptic neurone and provides an important pathway for the metabolism of monoamines; thus, MAOIs inhibit the metabolism of monoamines, resulting in an accumulation of amine neurotransmitters within the synapse.

b) Indications

1. Treatment of atypical depressive disorders with anxiety, phobic anxiety, obsessional, hysterical or hypochondrical symptoms (i.e. neurotic symptoms).

2. Treatment of resistant depression (particularly tranylcypromine – but it carries a risk of dependence because of its amphetamine-like action).

3. Treatment of anxiety neuroses – some evidence for usefulness in panic disorders due to anxiolytic properties.

4. Treatment of phobic anxiety neuroses – reduce agoraphobic symptoms, but there is a high relapse rate when drugs are stopped.

c) Adverse effects

1. Potentiate the pressor effect of tyramine and dopa present in certain foods (e.g. Chianti wine, cheese spreads, well-hung game, pickled herring, banana skins, broad bean 'pods', marmite and bovril).

2. Potentiate the pressor effect of indirect-acting sympathomimetic drugs (e.g. proprietary cough mixtures, nasal decongestants, anaesthetics).
   N.B. both of these types of interaction may cause a dangerous rise in blood pressure ('hypertensive crisis') with fatal consequences; an early warning sign may be a throbbing headache.

3. TCAs, second-generation antidepressants and SSRIs, should not be started until 2 weeks after MAOIs have been stopped in view of the persistence of the effects of MAOIs following discontinuation.

4. MAOIs should not be started until one week after TCAs and second-generation antidepressants have been stopped.

5. MAOIs should not be started until 2 weeks after SSRIs have been stopped with the exception of fluoxetine (see below).

6. MAOIs should not be started until 5 weeks after fluoxetine has been stopped in view of its long half-life and active metabolite (norfluoxetine).

7. The most commonly prescribed MAOI is phenelzine; however, MAOIs are the least commonly prescribed of the antidepressant drugs because:

   i) They interact dangerously with certain foods and drugs (see above).

   ii) The washout period following MAOI discontinuation is 2 weeks – cf. the washout period of one week following discontinuation of TCAs and second-generation antidepressants (see above).

   iii) The main indication for MAOIs is atypical depressive disorders (see above), i.e. MAOIs are not generally indicated for endogenous depressive disorders with biological features of depression (except resistant cases when they may be combined with TCAs under specialist supervision).

V. REVERSIBLE INHIBITORS OF MONOAMINE OXIDASE TYPE A (RIMAs)

Moclobemide (the first RIMA) is due to be launched in the UK in 1993.

a) Mode of action

Selectively and reversibly inhibit monoamine oxidase type A. In contrast, conventional MAOIs inhibit monoamine oxidase types A and B and are irreversible.
The antidepressant effect of MAOIs is considered to be a result of inhibition of monoamine oxidase type A.

b) Indications

1. Treatment of depressive disorders (endogenous and atypical).
2. May also be useful in anxiety neuroses and phobic anxiety neuroses (e.g. social phobias).

c) Adverse effects

RIMAs do potentiate the pressor effect of tyramine and dopa-containing foods, and indirect-acting sympathomimetic drugs, although the interaction is thought to be less than with conventional MAOIs.

VI. THYROXINE

Indications

1. It may be used to augment antidepressant drug treatment in resistant depression.

2. It may have mood elevating properties when clinical depression and subclinical hypothyroidism co-exist (the latter being defined as a free thyroxine serum level at the lower end of the normal range).

CHAPTER 4

Mood Stabilizers

I. LITHIUM CARBONATE

a) Mode of action

The precise mechanism by which lithium produces its therapeutic effect is complex and poorly understood.

Mechanism of therapeutic effects:

1. Decreased neurotransmitter postsynaptic receptor sensitivity.

2. Stimulates exit of Na^+ from cells where intracellular Na^+ is elevated (as in depression) by stimulating the Na^+/K^+ pump mechanism.

3. Stimulates entry of Na^+ into cells where intracellular Na^+ is reduced (as in mania).

4. Influences Ca^{2+} and Na^+ transfer across cell membranes including the Ca^{2+}-dependent release of neurotransmitter.

5. Inhibits adenyl cyclase necessary for the conversion of ATP to cyclic AMP – this mechanism mediates the long-term side-effects of nephrogenic diabetes insipidus and hypothyroidism (see below), i.e. lithium blocks ADH-sensitive adenyl cyclase and TSH-sensitive adenyl cyclase respectively.

6. Interacts with Ca^{2+} and Mg^{2+}, thereby increasing cell membrane permeability.

b) Indications

1. Treatment of depressive disorders:

   i) Treatment can be justified in the acute stages of depressive disorders, when other measures have failed.

   ii) Effective in patients who have failed to respond to a cyclic antidepressant drug (mono-, bi-, tri- or tetracyclic antidepressants), i.e. effective in resistant depression.

   iii) Enhances the effects of TCAs and MAOIs.

   iv) Enhances the effects of SSRIs – however, lithium should be introduced cautiously because of the risk of NMS developing (due to enhanced serotonergic activity); this risk appears to be lowest with fluvoxamine.

2. Preventing relapse of depressive disorders:

   i) In unipolar affective disorders:

      - Lithium reduces the rate of relapse (but is probably no more effective than continuing TCA treatment).
      - After the first episode, treatment should be prolonged for 6 months post-clinical recovery.
      - After 2 or more episodes – treatment should be prolonged for several (1–3) years post-clinical recovery; lithium is particularly useful in the prophylaxis of recurrent unipolar depression.
      - Continuing treatment with lithium reduces the rate of relapse after treatment with ECT.

ii) In bipolar affective disorders – prolonged administration of lithium (5 years) prevents relapses into depression.

3. Treatment of mania:

   Lithium is effective in high doses (1000 mg nocte), but the therapeutic response usually only occurs in the second week of treatment; thus, the response to lithium is slower than the response to antipsychotic drugs.

4. Preventing relapse of mania:

   In bipolar affective disorders, prolonged administration of lithium (5 years) prevents relapses into mania.

5. Treatment of mixed affective states.

6. Prophylaxis of schizoaffective disorders – in combination with an antipsychotic depot injection.

7. Treatment of aggressive or self-mutilating behaviour.

c) Adverse effects

1. Short-term side-effects:

   i) Gastrointestinal disturbances (nausea, vomiting, diarrhoea).
   ii) Fine tremor.
   iii) Muscle weakness.
   iv) Polyuria.
   v) Polydypsia.

2. Long-term side-effects:

   i) Nephrogenic diabetes insipidus.
   ii) Hypothyroidism.
   iii) Cardiotoxicity.
   iv) Irreversible renal damage.
   v) Oedema.
   vi) Weight gain.
   vii) Poor short-term memory
   viii) Tardive dyskinesia and other movement disorders.

3. Toxic effects:

   i) Increasing gastrointestinal disturbances (anorexia, vomiting, diarrhoea).

   ii) Increasing CNS disturbances (coarse tremor, drowsiness, ataxia, nystagmus, incoordination, slurring of speech, convulsions, coma).

   iii) The effects of lithium overdosage may be fatal – hence it is important that the serum lithium level be closely monitored to ensure that it lies within the therapeutic range of 0.4 – 1.0 mmol/L (the lower end of this range is for maintenance therapy; the higher end of this range is for treatment in the acute stages of illness) on blood samples taken 12 hours after the last dose of lithium; serum lithium levels over 1.5 mmol/L may be fatal.

   iv) Once stabilized on lithium carbonate, the following should be monitored:

- Every 3 months – serum lithium level and serum urea and electrolytes.
- Every 6 months – thyroid functions test.
- Every 12 months – ECG.

N.B. Before commencing lithium therapy, baseline investigations should include a serum urea and electrolytes, a thyroid function test and an ECG.

4. Drug interactions:

   i) Sodium depletion raises the serum lithium level and may result in lithium toxicity – therefore the concurrent use of diuretics (particularly thiazides) should be avoided.

   ii) The concurrent use of carbamazepine with lithium may result in neurotoxicity without raising the serum lithium level – hence if carbamazepine is added to lithium, it should be done so with caution – cf. the concurrent use of sodium valproate with lithium which is safe.

5. Contraindications:

   i) Pregnancy.
   ii) Breast feeding.
   iii) Renal impairment.

II. CARBAMAZEPINE

a) Mode of action

1. Structurally similar to the tricyclic antidepressant imipramine – however, carbamazepine has no effect on monoamine re-uptake.

2. Thought to mediate its therapeutic effect by inhibiting kindling phenomena in the limbic system.

b) Indications

1. Treatment of depressive disorders – treatment of resistant depression, i.e. worth a trial in patients who have failed to respond to a cyclic antidepressant drug and lithium carbonate.

2. Preventing relapse of depressive disorders:

   i) It prevents relapses into depression in both recurrent unipolar affective disorders and recurrent bipolar affective disorders.
   ii) It is the mood stabilizer of choice in patients with both epilepsy and bipolar affective disorder since it also has anticonvulsant properties.

3. Treatment of mania – carbamazepine is effective in high doses (400 mg t.d.s.), but the therapeutic response usually only occurs in the second week of treatment; thus, the response to carbamazepine is slower than the response to antipsychotic drugs.

4. Preventing relapse of mania:

   i) In patients who fail to respond to lithium carbonate – carbamazepine can either be substituted for or added to lithium; the two drugs appear to have a synergistic effect when used in combination (but see earlier note on their concurrent use).
   ii) In patients with the rapid-cycling form of bipolar affective disorder (i.e. 4 or more affective

episodes per year) – carbamazepine is a better prophylactic agent than lithium carbonate.

5. Treatment of all forms of epilepsy – except absence seizures.

6. Treatment of trigeminal neuralgia.

7. Treatment of behavioural disorders secondary to limbic epileptic instability.

8. Treatment of aggressive behaviour (including after head injury).

9. Treatment of acute alcohol withdrawal.

c) Adverse effects

1. Side-effects:

   i) Dizziness and drowsiness.
   ii) Generalized erythematous rash (3%).
   iii) Visual disturbances (especially double vision).
   iv) Gastrointestinal disturbances (anorexia, constipation).
   v) Leucopenia and other blood disorders.

2. Carbamazepine is initiated at a dosage of 200 mg b.d. and increased after one week to the usual therapeutic dosage of 200 mg t.d.s. required for prophylaxis (some patients may require 200 mg q.d.s.) – carbamazepine is a less toxic drug than lithium carbonate and regular serum level estimation appears to be unnecessary; however, because of the slight risk of leucopenia and other blood disorders, it is important that full blood count is monitored periodically.

III. SODIUM VALPROATE

a) Mode of action

Thought to mediate its therapeutic effect through indirect effects on GABA-ergic systems (i.e. it is a GABA-agonist), implicating a possible underlying biochemical disturbance of GABA deficiency in some affective disorders.

b) Indications

1. Treatment of depressive disorders – treatment of resistant depression, i.e. worth a trial in patients who have failed to respond to a cyclic antidepressant drug, lithium carbonate and carbamazepine.

2. Preventing relapse of depressive disorders – it prevents relapses into depression in bipolar affective disorders.

3. Treatment of mania – sodium valproate is effective in high doses (400 mg t.d.s.), but the therapeutic response usually only occurs in the second week of treatment; thus, the response to sodium valproate is slower than the response to antipsychotic drugs.

4. Preventing relapse of mania:

    i) Effective as a mood stabilizer in some manic patients who fail to respond to lithium carbonate and carbamazepine.
    ii) In the case of lithium carbonate, sodium valproate can be safely added to it and has been shown to enhance the effectiveness of lithium as a mood stabilizer.

5. Treatment of all forms of epilepsy.

c) Adverse effects

1. Side-effects.

   i) Recent concern over severe hepatic and pancreatic toxicity.
   ii) Haematological disturbance (thrombocytopenia, inhibition of platelet aggregation).

2. Sodium valproate is initiated at a dosage of 200 mg b.d. and increased after one week to the usual therapeutic dosage of 200 mg t.d.s. required for prophylaxis (some patients may require 200 mg q.d.s.) – sodium valproate is a less toxic drug than lithium and regular serum level estimation appears to be unnecessary; however, because of the slight risk of severe hepatic toxicity, severe pancreatic toxicity and haematological disturbance of platelet function, it is important that liver function tests, serum amylase level and full blood count are monitored periodically.